BAROTRAUMA

UNDERSTANDING CAUSES, DIAGNOSIS, TREATMENT, AND PREVENTION

DR. J.P JUDE

Table of Contents

CHAPTER ONE

Introduction

Barotrauma refers to injuries caused by changes in pressure between a gas-filled space inside the body and the surrounding environment. It commonly occurs during activities such as scuba diving, flying in an aircraft, or traveling to high altitudes. Barotrauma can affect various parts of the body, including the ears, sinuses, lungs, and gastrointestinal system, leading to a range of symptoms and complications. Understanding the causes, risk factors, and preventive measures for barotrauma is essential for minimizing the risk of injury and ensuring safety during pressure-related activities.

Types of Barotrauma:

Ear Barotrauma:

Eustachian Tube Dysfunction: Inability to equalize pressure between the middle ear and the environment, leading to discomfort, pain, fullness, or hearing loss.

Middle Ear Barotrauma: Injury to the middle ear due to pressure changes, causing ear pain, tinnitus (ringing in the ears), or ear drum rupture.

Sinus Barotrauma:

Sinus Squeeze: Pain or discomfort in the sinus cavities due to pressure changes, leading to sinus congestion, facial pain, or headaches.

Lung Barotrauma:

Pulmonary Barotrauma: Lung injury caused by rapid changes in pressure, leading to air trapping, pneumothorax (collapsed lung), or arterial gas embolism.

Gastrointestinal Barotrauma:

Abdominal Squeeze: Injury to the gastrointestinal tract due to pressure changes, causing abdominal pain, bloating, or discomfort.

Common Causes of Barotrauma:

Scuba Diving:

Descending and Ascending: Rapid changes in pressure while descending or ascending during scuba diving can lead to ear and lung barotrauma.

Flying in Aircraft:

Takeoff and Landing: Pressure changes during takeoff and landing can cause ear and sinus barotrauma due to the rapid changes in cabin pressure.

High Altitude Activities:

Mountain Climbing and Skydiving: Exposure to high altitudes without proper acclimatization and pressure adjustments can lead to lung and sinus barotrauma.

Hyperbaric Oxygen Therapy:

Medical Treatment: Exposure to high-pressure oxygen environments during hyperbaric oxygen therapy can cause lung and ear barotrauma if pressure is not regulated properly.

Risk Factors for Barotrauma:

Anatomical Factors: Narrow or obstructed Eustachian tubes, sinus congestion, or lung conditions may increase susceptibility to barotrauma.

Medical Conditions: Respiratory infections, allergies, sinusitis, or previous ear or lung injuries can predispose individuals to barotrauma.

Behavioral Factors: Inadequate equalization techniques, rapid ascent or descent, improper pressure adjustments, or failure to follow safety guidelines during pressure-related activities can increase the risk of barotrauma.

Prevention Strategies for Barotrauma:

Equalization Techniques: Learn and practice proper equalization techniques, such as swallowing, yawning, or using the Valsalva maneuver, to equalize pressure in the ears and sinuses during pressure changes.

Pressure Adjustments: Gradually ascend or descend, make slow and controlled pressure adjustments, and follow recommended dive tables or altitude guidelines to minimize pressure differentials.

Medical Evaluation: Undergo a pre-activity medical evaluation, consult with healthcare professionals, and ensure medical clearance for pressure-related activities, especially if you have underlying medical conditions or risk factors for barotrauma.

Safety Guidelines: Adhere to safety guidelines, receive proper training, use appropriate equipment, and follow established protocols for scuba diving, flying, high altitude activities, and hyperbaric oxygen therapy to reduce the risk of barotrauma.

Awareness and Monitoring: Be aware of symptoms, monitor for signs of barotrauma, and seek prompt medical attention if you experience discomfort, pain, or symptoms of pressure-related injuries during or after pressure-related activities.

Barotrauma is a potential risk during pressure-related activities and environments, requiring awareness, caution, and proper precautions to prevent injury and ensure safety. Understanding the types, causes, risk factors, and prevention strategies for barotrauma is essential for minimizing risks, promoting safety, and enjoying pressure-related activities responsibly.

If you participate in scuba diving, flying, high altitude activities, or hyperbaric oxygen therapy, consult with healthcare professionals, receive proper training, follow safety guidelines, and practice preventive measures to reduce the risk of barotrauma, protect your health, and enhance your overall well-being during pressure-related adventures and experiences.

Anatomy and Physiology Related to Barotrauma

Understanding the anatomy and physiology related to barotrauma is crucial for recognizing the mechanisms underlying pressure-related injuries and implementing effective preventive measures and management strategies. Barotrauma primarily affects the body's air-containing spaces, including the ears, sinuses, lungs, and gastrointestinal tract, where pressure differentials can lead to tissue damage, discomfort, and dysfunction. Here's an overview of the relevant anatomy and physiology associated with barotrauma:

Ear Anatomy and Physiology:

Middle Ear:

Eustachian Tube: Connects the middle ear to the nasopharynx, equalizing pressure between the middle ear and the external environment by allowing air to flow in and out.

Tympanic Membrane (Eardrum): Separates the outer ear from the middle ear, transmitting sound vibrations and protecting the middle ear from external contaminants.

Inner Ear:

Cochlea: Converts sound vibrations into electrical signals transmitted to the brain for interpretation.

Vestibular System: Maintains balance and spatial orientation, consisting of semicircular canals and otolithic organs.

Sinus Anatomy and Physiology:

Paranasal Sinuses: Air-filled cavities in the skull connected to the nasal passages, reducing skull weight, resonating voice, and producing mucus to moisten and filter air.

Sinus Ostia: Openings connecting the sinuses to the nasal passages, allowing air and mucus exchange and equalizing pressure between the sinuses and the external environment.

Lung Anatomy and Physiology:

Respiratory Tract: Includes the airways (trachea, bronchi, bronchioles) and alveoli, where gas exchange (oxygen and carbon dioxide) occurs.

Diaphragm and Intercostal Muscles: Primary muscles of respiration, facilitating inhalation and exhalation by changing thoracic volume and creating pressure differentials.

Gastrointestinal Anatomy and Physiology:

Gastrointestinal Tract: Includes the esophagus, stomach, and intestines, responsible for digestion, absorption, and elimination of food and waste products.

Abdominal Cavity: Houses the gastrointestinal organs, liver, spleen, and other structures, maintaining intra-abdominal pressure and protecting internal organs.

Physiology of Barotrauma:

Pressure Changes:

Gas Laws: Boyle's Law states that the pressure of a gas is inversely proportional to its volume ($P1V1 = P2V2$), meaning that as volume decreases (e.g., during descent), pressure increases, and vice versa (e.g., during ascent).

Equalization Mechanisms:

Eustachian Tube Function: Equalizes pressure between the middle ear and the external environment by opening and closing to allow air flow, preventing pressure differentials and barotrauma.

CHAPTER TWO

Sinus Drainage: Facilitates mucus drainage and equalizes pressure between the sinuses and nasal passages to prevent sinus barotrauma.

Gas Exchange and Expansion:

Lung Compliance: Lung expansion and contraction during inhalation and exhalation, maintaining gas exchange and accommodating pressure changes without tissue damage.

Alveolar Capillary Barrier: Protects against gas embolism and pulmonary barotrauma by filtering and regulating gas exchange in the alveoli.

Tissue Protection and Adaptation:

Adaptation to Pressure Changes: Gradual adaptation and acclimatization to pressure changes during diving, flying, or high-altitude activities, allowing tissues to adjust and preventing barotrauma.

Barotrauma involves complex interactions between anatomy and physiology, where pressure changes and equalization mechanisms play a critical role in protecting air-containing spaces and preventing tissue damage. Understanding the anatomical structures involved, physiological responses to pressure changes, and mechanisms of equalization and adaptation is essential for recognizing risk factors, implementing preventive measures, and managing barotrauma effectively during pressure-related activities and environments.

If you engage in scuba diving, flying, high-altitude activities, or hyperbaric oxygen therapy, familiarize yourself with the anatomy and physiology related to barotrauma, learn proper equalization techniques, and follow safety guidelines to minimize risks, protect your health, and enjoy pressure-related experiences safely and responsibly. Safety awareness, knowledge, and proactive management are key to preventing barotrauma, ensuring well-being, and promoting a healthier and safer exploration of pressure-related adventures and challenges.

Types and Causes of Barotrauma

Barotrauma encompasses various types of injuries caused by changes in pressure between a gas-filled space inside the body and the surrounding environment. These pressure differentials can lead to tissue damage, discomfort, and dysfunction in the ears, sinuses, lungs, and gastrointestinal tract. Understanding the different types and underlying causes of barotrauma is essential for recognizing risk factors, implementing preventive measures, and managing potential injuries effectively. Here's an overview of the types and causes of barotrauma:

Types of Barotrauma:

Ear Barotrauma:

Middle Ear Barotrauma: Injury to the middle ear due to pressure changes, causing ear pain, tinnitus (ringing in the ears), or ear drum rupture.

Eustachian Tube Dysfunction: Inability to equalize pressure between the middle ear and the external environment, leading to discomfort, pain, fullness, or hearing loss.

Inner Ear Barotrauma: Pressure-related injuries to the inner ear structures, affecting balance and hearing.

Sinus Barotrauma:

Sinus Squeeze: Pain or discomfort in the sinus cavities due to pressure changes, leading to sinus congestion, facial pain, or headaches.

Aerosinusitis: Inflammation of the sinuses caused by pressure changes during flying or diving, leading to sinus pain, congestion, and inflammation.

Lung Barotrauma:

Pulmonary Barotrauma: Lung injury caused by rapid changes in pressure, leading to air trapping, pneumothorax (collapsed lung), or arterial gas embolism.

Barotrauma-Induced Pneumothorax: Accumulation of air in the pleural space due to lung rupture, causing chest pain, shortness of breath, and respiratory distress.

Gastrointestinal Barotrauma:

Abdominal Squeeze: Injury to the gastrointestinal tract due to pressure changes, causing abdominal pain, bloating, or discomfort.

Gas Embolism: Introduction of gas bubbles into the bloodstream, leading to vascular occlusion, tissue ischemia, and organ damage.

Common Causes of Barotrauma:

Scuba Diving:

Descending and Ascending: Rapid changes in pressure while descending or ascending during scuba diving can lead to ear and lung barotrauma.

Improper Equalization: Failure to equalize pressure in the ears, sinuses, or mask can result in barotrauma during diving.

Flying in Aircraft:

Takeoff and Landing: Pressure changes during takeoff and landing can cause ear and sinus barotrauma due to the rapid changes in cabin pressure.

Air Travel with Respiratory Infections: Flying with sinus congestion, cold, or respiratory infections can increase susceptibility to ear and sinus barotrauma.

High Altitude Activities:

Mountain Climbing and Skydiving: Exposure to high altitudes without proper acclimatization and pressure adjustments can lead to lung and sinus barotrauma.

Rapid Ascent or Descent: Rapid changes in altitude without proper acclimatization and gradual pressure adjustments can result in barotrauma.

Hyperbaric Oxygen Therapy:

Medical Treatment: Exposure to high-pressure oxygen environments during hyperbaric oxygen therapy can cause lung and ear barotrauma if pressure is not regulated properly.

Oxygen Toxicity: Prolonged exposure to high concentrations of oxygen can lead to oxygen toxicity, resulting in lung and central nervous system damage.

Risk Factors for Barotrauma:

Anatomical Factors: Narrow or obstructed Eustachian tubes, sinus congestion, or lung conditions may increase susceptibility to barotrauma.

Medical Conditions: Respiratory infections, allergies, sinusitis, or previous ear or lung injuries can predispose individuals to barotrauma.

Behavioral Factors: Inadequate equalization techniques, rapid ascent or descent, improper pressure adjustments, or failure to follow safety guidelines during pressure-related activities can increase the risk of barotrauma.

Barotrauma involves a range of injuries affecting the ears, sinuses, lungs, and gastrointestinal tract due to pressure changes in the surrounding environment. Recognizing the types, causes, and risk factors for barotrauma is essential for implementing preventive measures, practicing proper equalization techniques, and seeking prompt medical attention when experiencing symptoms of pressure-related injuries. Whether engaging in scuba diving, flying, high-altitude activities, or hyperbaric oxygen therapy, understanding the potential risks and adopting safe practices are key to minimizing the risk of barotrauma, protecting your health, and enjoying pressure-related experiences safely and responsibly. Safety awareness, knowledge, and proactive management are essential for preventing barotrauma, ensuring well-being, and promoting a healthier and safer exploration of pressure-related adventures and challenges.

Risk Factors for Barotrauma

Barotrauma occurs due to changes in pressure between a gas-filled space inside the body and the surrounding environment, leading to tissue damage, discomfort, and dysfunction in various body areas such as the ears, sinuses, lungs, and gastrointestinal tract. Understanding the risk factors associated with barotrauma is essential for identifying individuals who may be more susceptible to pressure-related injuries and implementing preventive measures to minimize the risk of complications. Here's an overview of the common risk factors for barotrauma:

Anatomical Factors:

Narrow or Obstructed Eustachian Tubes:

Eustachian Tube Dysfunction: Difficulty in equalizing pressure between the middle ear and the external environment, increasing the risk of middle ear barotrauma during pressure changes.

Sinus Congestion or Blockage:

Sinusitis: Inflammation or infection of the sinuses, obstructing sinus ostia and increasing susceptibility to sinus barotrauma.

Nasal Polyps or Deviated Septum: Structural abnormalities in the nasal passages and sinuses can hinder proper equalization and drainage, predisposing to barotrauma.

Lung Conditions:

Chronic Obstructive Pulmonary Disease (COPD): Reduced lung function and compliance can increase vulnerability to lung barotrauma during pressure changes.

Asthma: Bronchial hyperreactivity and airway inflammation may exacerbate lung barotrauma under pressure-related conditions.

Medical Conditions:

Respiratory Infections:

Cold, Flu, or Upper Respiratory Infections: Inflammation and congestion of the respiratory tract can impair equalization and increase susceptibility to ear and sinus barotrauma.

Allergies:

Seasonal Allergies or Hay Fever: Nasal congestion, mucosal swelling, and increased mucus production can obstruct sinus ostia and elevate the risk of sinus barotrauma.

Previous Ear or Lung Injuries:

History of Barotrauma: Previous episodes of barotrauma or injuries to the ears, sinuses, or lungs can indicate increased susceptibility to recurrent pressure-related injuries.

Behavioral Factors:

Inadequate Equalization Techniques:

Improper Equalization: Failure to effectively equalize pressure in the ears, sinuses, or mask during diving, flying, or altitude changes can predispose to barotrauma.

Rapid Ascent or Descent:

Uncontrolled Pressure Changes: Rapid changes in altitude or depth without proper acclimatization, gradual ascent or descent, and pressure adjustments can lead to barotrauma.

Failure to Follow Safety Guidelines:

Non-Adherence to Safety Protocols: Ignoring safety guidelines, skipping pre-dive or pre-flight checks, or neglecting proper equipment use and maintenance can increase the risk of barotrauma.

Other Risk Factors:

Age:

Children and Infants: Immature Eustachian tubes and smaller airways may increase susceptibility to ear and lung barotrauma in younger individuals.

Underlying Medical Conditions:

Cardiovascular Diseases: Heart conditions affecting blood circulation and oxygenation may exacerbate the effects of barotrauma and increase the risk of complications.

Neurological Disorders: Conditions affecting neurological function and sensory perception may impair equalization techniques and increase vulnerability to barotrauma.

Identifying and understanding the risk factors for barotrauma is crucial for assessing individual susceptibility, implementing preventive measures, and promoting safe practices during pressure-related activities and environments. Whether engaging in scuba diving, flying, high-altitude activities, or hyperbaric oxygen therapy, recognizing the potential risks and adopting appropriate precautions are key to minimizing the risk of barotrauma, protecting your health, and ensuring a safer and more enjoyable experience. Safety awareness, knowledge, and proactive management are essential for preventing barotrauma, maintaining well-being, and promoting a healthier and safer exploration of pressure-related adventures and challenges.

Clinical Presentation of Barotrauma

Barotrauma presents with a range of clinical symptoms and signs depending on the affected anatomical structures and the severity of the pressure-related injuries. Recognizing the clinical presentation of barotrauma is essential for timely diagnosis, appropriate management, and prevention of complications. Here's an overview of the common clinical presentations associated with different types of barotrauma:

Ear Barotrauma:

Middle Ear Barotrauma:

Ear Pain: Sharp, stabbing, or aching pain in one or both ears.

Hearing Loss: Temporary or permanent hearing impairment or muffled hearing.

Tinnitus: Ringing, buzzing, or roaring sounds in the ears (subjective tinnitus).

Eustachian Tube Dysfunction:

Ear Fullness or Pressure: Sensation of fullness, pressure, or blockage in the ears.

Hearing Difficulty: Difficulty hearing or muffled sounds.

Dizziness or Vertigo: Sensation of spinning, lightheadedness, or imbalance.

Inner Ear Barotrauma:

Vertigo: Episodes of dizziness, spinning, or loss of balance.

Nausea and Vomiting: Accompanying symptoms with severe vertigo.

Hearing Loss: Sudden or gradual hearing loss.

Tinnitus: Ringing, buzzing, or hissing sounds in the ears.

Sinus Barotrauma:

Sinus Squeeze:

Facial Pain or Pressure: Pain or pressure in the sinus areas (forehead, cheeks, or around the eyes).

Headache: Tension-type headache or sinus headache.

CHAPTER THREE

Nasal Congestion: Blocked or stuffy nose.

Mucus Discharge: Clear or bloody nasal discharge.

Aerosinusitis:

Severe Facial Pain: Sharp, intense pain in the sinus areas.

Nasal Bleeding: Epistaxis or bloody discharge from the nose.

Sinus Inflammation: Redness, swelling, or tenderness over the sinuses.

Lung Barotrauma:

Pulmonary Barotrauma:

Chest Pain: Sharp, stabbing, or squeezing chest pain.

Shortness of Breath: Difficulty breathing or breathlessness.

Cough: Dry or productive cough.

Hemoptysis: Coughing up blood or bloody sputum.

Respiratory Distress: Rapid breathing, wheezing, or cyanosis (blue discoloration of the lips and skin).

Gastrointestinal Barotrauma:

Abdominal Squeeze:

Abdominal Pain: Cramping, sharp, or dull pain in the abdomen.

Bloating or Distension: Feeling of fullness, bloating, or abdominal swelling.

Nausea and Vomiting: Nausea, vomiting, or gastrointestinal discomfort.

Neurological and Systemic Symptoms:

Central Nervous System Involvement:

Dizziness or Vertigo: Sensation of spinning, lightheadedness, or imbalance.

Confusion or Disorientation: Altered mental status or cognitive impairment.

Seizures: Uncontrolled muscle contractions, twitching, or loss of consciousness.

Barotrauma can manifest with a variety of clinical symptoms and signs affecting the ears, sinuses, lungs, gastrointestinal tract, and central nervous system. Recognizing the clinical presentation of barotrauma, conducting a thorough medical evaluation, and performing appropriate diagnostic tests (e.g., physical examination, otoscopy, tympanometry, imaging studies) are essential for accurate diagnosis, timely intervention, and effective management of pressure-related injuries.

If you or someone you know experiences symptoms of barotrauma during or after pressure-related activities such as scuba diving, flying, high-altitude activities, or hyperbaric oxygen therapy, seek prompt medical attention, consult with healthcare professionals, and follow recommended treatment guidelines to prevent complications, promote healing, and ensure a safer and healthier recovery. Safety awareness, knowledge, and proactive management are key to preventing barotrauma, maintaining well-being, and enjoying pressure-related experiences safely and responsibly.

Evaluation and Diagnosis of Barotrauma

Evaluation and diagnosis of barotrauma involve a comprehensive assessment of clinical symptoms, physical examination findings, and diagnostic tests to identify the affected anatomical structures and determine the severity of pressure-related injuries. Prompt and accurate diagnosis is essential for initiating appropriate treatment interventions, preventing complications, and promoting recovery. Here's an overview of the evaluation and diagnostic approach for barotrauma:

Clinical Evaluation:

Medical History:

Detailed History Taking: Inquire about recent exposure to pressure changes (e.g., diving, flying, high-altitude activities), onset and duration of symptoms, previous episodes of barotrauma, underlying medical conditions, and medications.

Symptom Assessment: Evaluate the presence, location, severity, and progression of symptoms related to ear, sinus, lung, gastrointestinal, and neurological involvement.

Physical Examination:

Otolaryngological Examination: Inspect the ears, nose, and throat; assess for signs of ear drum rupture, nasal congestion, sinus tenderness, and oropharyngeal abnormalities.

Pulmonary Examination: Auscultate lung sounds, assess respiratory rate, and check for signs of respiratory distress, such as wheezing, crackles, diminished breath sounds, or cyanosis.

Abdominal Examination: Palpate the abdomen for tenderness, distension, or organomegaly; assess bowel sounds and evaluate for signs of gastrointestinal involvement.

Diagnostic Tests:

Audiometric Testing:

Pure Tone Audiometry: Assess hearing acuity and identify potential hearing loss or abnormalities in the auditory system.

Imaging Studies:

Otoscopy: Examine the external ear canal and tympanic membrane for signs of inflammation, perforation, or injury.

Sinus X-rays or CT Scans: Evaluate sinus anatomy, identify sinus congestion, inflammation, or barotrauma-induced changes.

Chest X-ray or CT Scan: Assess lung parenchyma, pleural spaces, and identify signs of pneumothorax, lung collapse, or barotrauma-related lung injuries.

Pulmonary Function Tests:

Spirometry: Measure lung function parameters, assess respiratory mechanics, and identify obstructive or restrictive patterns suggestive of lung barotrauma.

Blood Gas Analysis:

Arterial Blood Gas (ABG) Analysis: Evaluate oxygenation, ventilation, and acid-base status to assess respiratory function and identify hypoxia or hypercapnia associated with lung barotrauma.

Gastrointestinal Evaluation:

Abdominal Ultrasound or CT Scan: Assess gastrointestinal anatomy, identify abdominal injuries, and evaluate for signs of gastrointestinal barotrauma or gas embolism.

Neurological Assessment:

Neurological Examination: Evaluate mental status, cranial nerve function, motor and sensory capabilities, reflexes, coordination, and balance to assess neurological involvement and identify central nervous system barotrauma.

The evaluation and diagnosis of barotrauma require a multidisciplinary approach involving detailed medical history, comprehensive physical examination, and targeted diagnostic testing to assess the extent and severity of pressure-related injuries affecting the ears, sinuses, lungs, gastrointestinal tract, and neurological system. Timely and accurate diagnosis facilitates appropriate treatment planning, symptom management, and preventive measures to minimize complications, promote recovery, and ensure a safer and healthier outcome for individuals experiencing barotrauma.

If you or someone you know exhibits symptoms suggestive of barotrauma following exposure to pressure changes, seek immediate medical attention, consult with healthcare professionals, and undergo a thorough evaluation to diagnose the condition, determine the underlying causes, and implement timely interventions tailored to individual needs, preferences, and health goals. Safety awareness, knowledge, and proactive management are essential for preventing barotrauma, ensuring well-being, and enjoying pressure-related experiences safely and responsibly.

Treatment approaches for barotrauma depend on the type, severity, and location of the pressure-related injuries affecting the ears, sinuses, lungs, gastrointestinal tract, and other anatomical structures. Prompt and appropriate treatment interventions are essential for managing symptoms, preventing complications, and promoting recovery. Here's an overview of the common treatment approaches for barotrauma:

Ear Barotrauma:

Middle Ear Barotrauma:

Watchful Waiting: Mild cases may resolve spontaneously with time and conservative management.

Pain Management: Over-the-counter pain relievers (e.g., acetaminophen, ibuprofen) or prescription analgesics for pain relief.

Otic Drops: Anti-inflammatory or antibiotic ear drops for symptomatic relief and prevention of infection.

Tympanostomy Tubes: Surgical placement of ventilation tubes in the eardrum for persistent middle ear effusion or recurrent barotrauma.

Eustachian Tube Dysfunction:

Autoinsufflation: Learn and practice proper equalization techniques to relieve pressure and promote Eustachian tube opening.

Decongestants: Oral or nasal decongestants (e.g., pseudoephedrine, oxymetazoline) to reduce nasal congestion and improve Eustachian tube function.

Nasal Steroids: Topical nasal corticosteroids (e.g., fluticasone, mometasone) to reduce mucosal inflammation and congestion.

Inner Ear Barotrauma:

Vestibular Rehabilitation: Physical therapy exercises to improve balance and reduce vertigo symptoms.

Medications: Antihistamines, anticholinergics, or benzodiazepines for symptomatic relief of vertigo, nausea, or dizziness.

Diuretics: Medications (e.g., acetazolamide) to reduce inner ear fluid volume and alleviate symptoms of Meniere's disease associated with inner ear barotrauma.

Sinus Barotrauma:

Sinus Squeeze:

Nasal Irrigation: Saline nasal sprays or irrigation (e.g., Neti pot) to clear nasal passages and relieve sinus pressure.

Topical Decongestants: Nasal decongestant sprays (e.g., oxymetazoline) for short-term relief of nasal congestion and sinus symptoms.

Antibiotics: Prescription antibiotics for bacterial sinusitis or secondary bacterial infections associated with sinus barotrauma.

Aerosinusitis:

Topical Steroids: Nasal corticosteroid sprays (e.g., fluticasone, mometasone) to reduce mucosal inflammation and nasal congestion.

Pain Management: Over-the-counter pain relievers or prescription analgesics for pain relief.

Nasal Oxygen Therapy: Supplemental oxygen therapy to alleviate sinus symptoms and promote healing.

Lung Barotrauma:

Pulmonary Barotrauma:

Oxygen Therapy: Supplemental oxygen to improve oxygenation and alleviate respiratory distress.

Chest Tube Placement: Insertion of a chest tube to evacuate air or fluid from the pleural space in cases of pneumothorax or pleural effusion.

Positive Pressure Ventilation: Mechanical ventilation support for severe respiratory failure or acute respiratory distress syndrome (ARDS) associated with lung barotrauma.

Gastrointestinal Barotrauma:

Abdominal Squeeze:

Symptomatic Management: Over-the-counter antacids, proton pump inhibitors, or H2 blockers for acid reflux, heartburn, or gastrointestinal discomfort.

Pain Management: Analgesics or antispasmodics for abdominal pain relief.

Observation and Monitoring: Close monitoring for signs of gastrointestinal complications, such as perforation, bleeding, or ischemia, requiring urgent medical intervention.

Neurological and Systemic Treatment:

Neurological Barotrauma:

Neurological Monitoring: Continuous neurological assessment and monitoring for signs of central nervous system involvement, such as altered mental status, seizures, or neurological deficits.

Antiepileptic Medications: Antiseizure medications (e.g., phenytoin, levetiracetam) for seizure control and management of barotrauma-induced seizures.

The treatment approaches for barotrauma involve a combination of conservative management, symptomatic relief, supportive care, and surgical interventions tailored to individual needs, symptoms, and severity of pressure-related injuries. Timely and appropriate treatment planning, multidisciplinary care, and close monitoring are essential for managing barotrauma effectively, preventing complications, promoting recovery, and ensuring a safer and healthier outcome for individuals experiencing pressure-related injuries.

If you or someone you know exhibits symptoms of barotrauma following exposure to pressure changes, seek immediate medical attention, consult with healthcare professionals, and undergo a thorough evaluation to diagnose the condition, determine the underlying causes, and implement timely interventions tailored to individual needs, preferences, and health goals. Safety awareness, knowledge, and proactive management are key to preventing barotrauma, maintaining well-being, and enjoying pressure-related experiences safely and responsibly.

Prevention Strategies for Barotrauma

Prevention strategies for barotrauma focus on reducing the risk of pressure-related injuries affecting the ears, sinuses, lungs, gastrointestinal tract, and other anatomical structures during exposure to pressure changes in various environments such as scuba diving, flying, high-altitude activities, or hyperbaric oxygen therapy. Adopting proactive measures, practicing proper techniques, and following safety guidelines are essential for minimizing the risk of barotrauma and ensuring a safer and more enjoyable experience. Here's an overview of the common prevention strategies for barotrauma:

CHAPTER FOUR

General Prevention Strategies:

Education and Awareness:

Knowledge of Pressure Changes: Understand the principles of pressure changes and their effects on the body during diving, flying, or altitude changes.

Safety Briefings and Training: Attend safety briefings, training sessions, or educational programs on barotrauma prevention, risk factors, and emergency procedures.

Proper Equalization Techniques:

Ear Equalization: Learn and practice effective equalization techniques (e.g., Valsalva maneuver, Toynbee maneuver, Frenzel maneuver) to equalize pressure in the ears and prevent middle ear barotrauma during scuba diving, flying, or altitude changes.

Sinus Equalization: Perform gentle nasal blowing or swallowing to equalize pressure in the sinuses and prevent sinus barotrauma during pressure changes.

Slow and Controlled Ascent/Descent:

Gradual Pressure Changes: Ascend or descend slowly and control the rate of pressure changes during diving, flying, or altitude activities to allow adequate time for equalization and prevent rapid pressure differentials leading to barotrauma.

Regular Health Check-ups:

Medical Evaluation: Undergo regular medical examinations, screenings, or consultations with healthcare professionals to assess fitness for diving, flying, or high-altitude activities and identify potential risk factors or contraindications for pressure-related environments.

Scuba Diving Prevention Strategies:

Pre-Dive Checks:

Equipment Inspection: Conduct thorough pre-dive checks of scuba gear, including regulators, masks, snorkels, and gauges, to ensure proper functioning and prevent equipment failure or malfunction leading to barotrauma.

Safety Protocols: Follow established safety protocols, guidelines, or buddy checks before, during, and after diving to ensure equipment readiness, proper equalization, and emergency preparedness.

Dive Planning and Monitoring:

Dive Profiles: Plan and monitor dive profiles, including depths, durations, and ascent rates, to adhere to safe diving practices, decompression limits, and prevent rapid pressure changes causing barotrauma.

Air Consumption: Monitor air consumption, maintain adequate buoyancy control, and practice controlled ascents to conserve air supply, avoid exertion, and reduce the risk of barotrauma during diving activities.

Flying and High-Altitude Prevention Strategies:

Pre-Flight Preparations:

Ear and Sinus Precautions: Use nasal decongestants or nasal sprays (e.g., oxymetazoline) prior to flying to reduce sinus congestion, improve Eustachian tube function, and facilitate equalization during ascent and descent.

Cabin Pressure: Choose flights with pressurized cabins, use specialized earplugs, or employ ear equalization techniques to manage pressure changes and minimize the risk of ear and sinus barotrauma during air travel.

Altitude Acclimatization:

Gradual Ascent: Acclimatize to high altitudes gradually, ascend slowly, and allow time for physiological adaptation to pressure changes to prevent altitude sickness, respiratory distress, or barotrauma-related complications during mountain climbing, hiking, or high-altitude activities.

Hyperbaric Oxygen Therapy Prevention Strategies:

Medical Screening and Monitoring:

Patient Assessment: Undergo comprehensive medical evaluations, screenings, or consultations with healthcare providers to assess eligibility, identify contraindications, and ensure safe and appropriate candidacy for hyperbaric oxygen therapy (HBOT) to minimize the risk of barotrauma and other potential complications.

Treatment Protocols and Monitoring:

Oxygen Delivery: Receive HBOT under controlled conditions, follow prescribed treatment protocols, and undergo continuous monitoring by trained professionals to regulate oxygen delivery, manage pressure changes, and prevent barotrauma-related injuries during hyperbaric treatments.

Prevention strategies for barotrauma involve a combination of education, awareness, proper techniques, equipment checks, safety protocols, and healthcare consultations tailored to specific pressure-related activities and environments. Implementing proactive measures, adhering to safety guidelines, and seeking professional guidance are essential for minimizing the risk of barotrauma, promoting safety, and ensuring a healthier and more enjoyable experience during pressure-related adventures and challenges.

If you engage in scuba diving, flying, high-altitude activities, or hyperbaric oxygen therapy, familiarize yourself with the prevention strategies, practice proper techniques, and follow safety recommendations to protect your health, reduce the risk of barotrauma, and enjoy pressure-related experiences safely and responsibly. Safety awareness, knowledge, and proactive management are key to preventing barotrauma, ensuring well-being, and promoting a healthier and safer exploration of pressure-related adventures and challenges.

Complications and Long-Term Effects

Barotrauma can lead to various complications and long-term effects depending on the severity of the pressure-related injuries, affected anatomical structures, and timely management of the condition. Recognizing potential complications, monitoring for long-term effects, and seeking appropriate medical care are essential for minimizing risks, preventing progression of injuries, and promoting recovery.

Here's an overview of the common complications and long-term effects associated with barotrauma:

Ear Barotrauma:

Chronic Otitis Media:

Persistent Middle Ear Inflammation: Chronic inflammation, recurrent infections, and fluid accumulation in the middle ear may lead to chronic otitis media, hearing loss, or tympanic membrane perforation requiring surgical intervention (e.g., tympanoplasty).

Inner Ear Damage:

Sensorineural Hearing Loss: Permanent hearing impairment or sensory neural hearing loss due to inner ear damage or cochlear injury from severe barotrauma.

Tinnitus:

Persistent Ringing or Buzzing: Chronic tinnitus or persistent ringing, buzzing, or hissing sounds in the ears may develop following inner ear damage or nerve irritation from barotrauma.

Sinus Barotrauma:

Chronic Sinusitis:

Persistent Sinus Inflammation: Chronic sinusitis, recurrent sinus infections, or sinus polyps may develop from persistent inflammation, mucosal damage, or obstruction of sinus ostia due to repeated sinus barotrauma.

Nasal Deformities:

Septal Deviation or Perforation: Nasal septal deviation, perforation, or nasal valve collapse may occur from repetitive sinus barotrauma, nasal trauma, or chronic inflammation affecting nasal structure and function.

Lung Barotrauma:

Pneumothorax:

Collapsed Lung: Spontaneous pneumothorax, tension pneumothorax, or recurrent pneumothorax may develop from lung barotrauma, alveolar rupture, or air leakage into the pleural space requiring chest tube placement or surgical intervention.

Pulmonary Fibrosis:

Interstitial Lung Disease: Chronic inflammation, fibrotic changes, or scarring of lung tissue may lead to interstitial lung disease, restrictive lung disorders, or impaired gas exchange following severe lung barotrauma or prolonged oxygen toxicity.

Gastrointestinal Barotrauma:

Gastroesophageal Reflux Disease (GERD):

Chronic Acid Reflux: Gastrointestinal reflux disease, esophageal inflammation, or Barrett's esophagus may develop from chronic acid reflux, esophageal irritation, or functional impairment of the lower esophageal sphincter due to gastrointestinal barotrauma.

Bowel Perforation:

Intestinal Injury: Bowel perforation, ischemia, or abdominal compartment syndrome may occur from severe abdominal barotrauma, gas embolism, or vascular occlusion affecting gastrointestinal integrity and function.

Neurological and Systemic Complications:

Central Nervous System Damage:

Neurological Deficits: Permanent neurological deficits, cognitive impairments, or sensory-motor dysfunction may result from central nervous system barotrauma, cerebral air embolism, or ischemic stroke due to gas embolism or vascular occlusion.

Oxygen Toxicity:

Seizures or Central Nervous System Effects: Prolonged exposure to high concentrations of oxygen during hyperbaric oxygen therapy may lead to oxygen toxicity, seizures, or central nervous system manifestations affecting brain function, sensory perception, or motor coordination.

Long-Term Effects and Quality of Life:

Quality of Life Impairment:

Functional Limitations: Persistent symptoms, physical impairments, or functional limitations affecting daily activities, social interactions, or occupational performance may result in reduced quality of life, psychological distress, or emotional well-being following unresolved or untreated barotrauma-related complications.

Psychological and Emotional Impact:

Anxiety, Depression, or Post-Traumatic Stress: Psychological trauma, anxiety disorders, depressive symptoms, or post-traumatic stress reactions may develop from traumatic experiences, chronic health issues, or long-term complications associated with barotrauma affecting mental health, emotional resilience, or psychosocial adjustment.

Barotrauma can lead to various complications, long-term effects, and quality of life impairments affecting physical health, mental well-being, and overall functional status. Recognizing potential risks, monitoring for complications, seeking timely medical care, and adopting preventive measures are essential for minimizing the impact of barotrauma, promoting recovery, and ensuring a healthier and safer outcome for individuals experiencing pressure-related injuries.

If you or someone you know exhibits symptoms of barotrauma, experiences complications, or faces long-term effects following exposure to pressure changes, seek immediate medical attention, consult with healthcare professionals, and undergo a thorough evaluation, diagnosis, and treatment planning tailored to individual needs, preferences, and health goals. Safety awareness, knowledge, and proactive management are key to preventing barotrauma, ensuring well-being, and promoting a healthier and safer exploration of pressure-related adventures and challenges.

Conclusion

In conclusion, barotrauma represents a complex and potentially serious medical condition resulting from pressure-related injuries affecting various anatomical structures such as the ears, sinuses, lungs, gastrointestinal tract, and central nervous system. Understanding the mechanisms, recognizing the risk factors, and implementing preventive measures are essential for minimizing the risk of barotrauma, ensuring safety, and promoting a healthier and more enjoyable experience during pressure-related activities and environments.

The evaluation, diagnosis, and management of barotrauma require a multidisciplinary approach involving detailed medical history, comprehensive physical examination, and targeted diagnostic testing to assess the extent and severity of pressure-related injuries. Timely and appropriate treatment interventions tailored to individual needs, symptoms, and severity of barotrauma are crucial for managing symptoms, preventing complications, and promoting recovery.

Prevention strategies for barotrauma involve a combination of education, awareness, proper techniques, equipment checks, safety protocols, and healthcare consultations tailored to specific pressure-related activities and environments. Implementing proactive measures, adhering to safety guidelines, and seeking professional guidance are essential for minimizing the risk of barotrauma, promoting safety, and ensuring a healthier and more enjoyable experience during pressure-related adventures and challenges.

Complications and long-term effects associated with barotrauma may include chronic inflammation, persistent symptoms, functional impairments, quality of life limitations, and psychological or emotional impact affecting physical health, mental well-being, and overall functional status. Recognizing potential risks, monitoring for complications, and seeking timely medical care are essential for minimizing the impact of barotrauma, promoting recovery, and ensuring a safer and healthier outcome for individuals experiencing pressure-related injuries.

If you or someone you know exhibits symptoms of barotrauma, experiences complications, or faces long-term effects following exposure to pressure changes, seek immediate medical attention, consult with healthcare professionals, and undergo a thorough evaluation, diagnosis, and treatment planning tailored to individual needs, preferences, and health goals. Safety awareness, knowledge, proactive management, and adherence to preventive measures are key to preventing barotrauma, maintaining well-being, and enjoying pressure-related experiences safely and responsibly.

Stay informed, be prepared, and prioritize safety to protect your health, reduce the risk of barotrauma, and enjoy pressure-related adventures and challenges responsibly, ensuring a healthier and safer exploration of exciting and rewarding experiences in various pressure environments. Your well-being, safety, and enjoyment are paramount, and proactive measures, informed decisions, and professional guidance are essential for navigating pressure-related activities and environments safely and responsibly.

THE END

9 798340 049780